THE ACID-ALKALINE DIET
Balancing the Body *Naturally*

Jo Stepaniak, MSEd

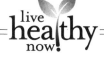

HEALTHY LIVING PUBLICATIONS
Summertown, Tennessee

© 2015 Jo Stepaniak

All rights reserved. No portion of this book may be reproduced by any means whatsoever, except for brief quotations in reviews, without written permission from the publisher.

Cover and interior design: Scattaregia Design

Healthy Living Publications,
a division of Book Publishing Company
PO Box 99
Summertown, TN 38483
888-260-8458
bookpubco.com

ISBN: 978-1-57067-332-0

Printed in the United States of America

20 19 18 17 16 15   1 2 3 4 5 6 7 8 9

Library of Congress Cataloging-in-Publication Data

Stepaniak, Jo,
The acid-alkaline diet : balancing the body naturally / Jo Stepaniak, MSEd.
    pages cm
ISBN 978-1-57067-332-0 (pbk.) -- ISBN 978-1-57067-862-2 (e-book)
1. Diet therapy. 2. Acid-base imbalances--Diet therapy. 3. Nutritionally induced diseases. I. Title.
RM216.S738 2015
615.8'54--dc23
                    2015026983

Printed on recycled paper

Book Publishing Company is a member of Green Press Initiative. We chose to print this title on paper with 100% post-consumer recycled content, processed without chlorine, which saved the following natural resources:

- 18 trees
- 563 pounds of solid waste
- 8,414 gallons of water
- 1,551 pounds of greenhouse gases
- 8 million BTUs of energy

For more information on Green Press Initiative, visit greenpressinitiative.org. Environmental impact estimates were made using the Environmental Defense Fund Paper Calculator. For more information, visit papercalculator.org.

> The information in this book is presented for educational purposes only. It isn't intended to be a substitute for the medical advice of a physician or other health care professional.

Contents

4	Introduction
4	Understanding pH
5	Acidosis and Alkalosis
12	The Effects of pH on the Environment and Our Food
13	The Effects of pH on Our Health
16	The Theory Behind the Acid-Alkaline Diet
23	Measuring the Acid and Alkaline Effects of Food
31	Improve Your pH Balance Naturally
34	Alkalizing Foods
35	Conclusion
35	Alkalizing Recipes
47	About the Author

Introduction

Using food to improve health isn't a new concept. In fact, Hippocrates, who was born around 460 BC and is considered the father of modern medicine, is credited with saying, "Let food be thy medicine and medicine be thy food." This famous slogan has inspired the birth of some very positive and health-promoting dietary approaches as well as others that are based on unproven theories and ideas that are dangerously out of step both with current scientific understanding and contemporary nutritional studies.

Nutrition is a complicated field that is continually evolving. Dietary recommendations are evolving as well, along with the comprehensive body of nutritional knowledge that has grown out of evidence-based research. Nevertheless, our endless desire to increase longevity, eradicate disease, lose weight, and enhance overall well-being has given rise to a plethora of food crazes and fad diets that are not necessarily rooted in science or derived from fact. Although some of these hold great promise for improved health, many are based on little more than wishful thinking. Which category does the acid-alkaline diet fall into?

Understanding pH

The acid-alkaline diet, formerly known as the alkaline-ash diet and currently also known as the alkaline diet or the alkaline-acid diet, is a cluster of dietary approaches based on the notion that the human body is designed to function optimally when body fluids (blood and urine) are at a particular pH level. Acid and alkaline (also called basic or base) are two extremes that describe chemicals in much the same way that hot and cold are two extremes that describe temperature. Mixing acids and alkalies can cancel out their extreme effects, which is comparable to how hot and cold water can regulate and equalize water temperature.

The pH scale measures how acidic or alkaline a substance is. The scale ranges from 0 to 14. A substance that is neither acidic nor basic is considered neutral. Solutions with a pH lower than 7 are said to be acidic, and solutions with a pH greater than 7 are said to be basic, or alkaline. Pure water has a pH of 7 and is therefore neutral. When chemicals are mixed with water, the resulting solution can become either acidic or alkaline. Vinegar and lemon juice are acidic substances, and when they are mixed with water, the water will become acidic. Likewise, when laundry detergents and ammonia, which are basic, are mixed with water, the water will become alkaline.

Chemicals that are very alkaline or very acidic are called "reactive" and can cause severe burns. For example, automobile battery acid is an acidic chemical that is highly reactive. Lye, which is found in many household drain cleaners, is a very alkaline chemical that is reactive.

The pH of substances can be measured by using certain indicators that change color depending on the acidity or alkalinity of the elements being tested. The color that is produced can then be compared with a standard color chart to measure the pH level to the nearest whole number. More precise and accurate measurements are possible if the color is measured with a spectrophotometer or colorimeter, which are instruments used for specifying colors in relation to other colors and measuring their relative intensities.

A "universal indicator" consists of a mixture of indicators that create a continuous color change from about pH 2 to pH 10. Universal indicator paper is made from absorbent, acid-free paper that has been impregnated with a universal indicator. Litmus, a substance used by alchemists in the Middle Ages and that is still readily available, is a naturally occurring pH indicator made from a mixture of lichen species, particularly *Roccella tinctoria*. The color changes to red in acid solutions and blue in alkaline solutions. The popular term "litmus test" is a widely used metaphor for any test that claims to authoritatively differentiate between alternatives.

Acidosis and Alkalosis

At the core of the acid-alkaline diet is the belief that most people's bodies are too acidic and that this creates an environment hostile to health and conducive to disease. Advocates of the diet contend that the ideal pH level of the human body is slightly alkaline, between 7.30 and 7.45, but that the average person's pH is far too acidic, between 5.5 and 6.5. Proponents state that this range has catastrophic effects on every system of the human body and, if left untreated, will interrupt all cellular activities and functions. But are these numbers realistic? Is there actually a single number that reflects the body's overall pH? Does the pH of various body fluids provide meaningful insights into our state of health? Can dietary changes and supplements truly affect the body's pH and prevent or reverse illness? The sections that follow will address and attempt to answer these questions.

Acidosis

When the body's fluids contain too much acid, this creates a condition known as acidosis. Acidosis occurs when the kidneys and lungs can't regulate the body's pH and keep it in balance. There are basically two types of acidosis: metabolic and respiratory. Metabolic acidosis occurs when the kidneys are unable to excrete acid buildup or when the body eliminates too much base. Respiratory acidosis occurs when the lungs do not properly eliminate carbon dioxide (an acid). When carbon dioxide builds up in the blood, the blood becomes more acidic. This type of acidosis is usually caused when the body is unable to remove enough carbon dioxide through breathing. Other names for respiratory acidosis are hypercapnic acidosis and carbon dioxide acidosis.

Acidosis is a serious clinical disturbance characterized by an increase in plasma acidity. In other words, the chemical balance of acids and alkalines in the blood gets off kilter. According to the *Merck Manual*, the etiology of metabolic acidosis is acid accumulation attributed to increased acid production or acid ingestion, decreased acid excretion, or specific gastrointestinal or renal losses. In laymen's terms, this condition occurs because the body is either making too much acid, isn't getting rid of enough acid, or doesn't have enough alkalines to offset the normal amount of acid. When this imbalance happens, chemical reactions and processes in the body don't function properly. Although severe acidosis can be life-threatening, some cases are mild. How the condition is treated depends on what's causing it.

Causes of Acidosis

A variety of factors can create an acid-base imbalance in the blood:

Hyperchloremic acidosis. Severe diarrhea, kidney problems, and overuse of laxatives can cause lower levels of bicarbonate, the alkaline that helps neutralize acids in the blood, and may result in hyperchloremic acidosis.

Ketoacidosis. When people with diabetes don't get enough insulin and become dehydrated, the body burns fat as fuel instead of carbohydrates, and this results in the production of substances known as ketones. An overabundance of ketones causes the blood to become acidic, a condition called ketoacidosis. Malnourishment (insufficient amounts of food over time) can also cause a buildup of ketones.

Lactic acidosis. Lactic acid can build up in the body when cells have insufficient oxygen, and this can lead to lactic acidosis. This condition can occur with cancer, cardiac arrest, extensive or serious infection, intense exercise, or severe drops in blood pressure. It can also be caused by medications (such as salicylates), MELAS (a very rare genetic mitochondrial disorder that affects energy production), seizures, or prolonged lack of oxygen from shock, heart failure, or severe anemia.

Renal tubular acidosis. When kidneys are healthy, they remove acid from the blood, and that acid is then excreted in the urine. Kidney diseases, a compromised immune system, and genetic disorders can damage the kidneys and impair this normal process, resulting in too much acid remaining in the blood and creating a condition known as renal tubular acidosis.

Respiratory acidosis. Lung disease and other respiratory ailments can cause a buildup of carbon dioxide in the body that results in blood that's too acidic. This condition is called respiratory acidosis.

Symptoms of Metabolic Acidosis

When the body is in a state of metabolic acidosis, the enzyme systems are running at maximum speed. This pushes the sympathetic nervous system beyond its normal limits and forces the adrenal glands into overdrive. Metabolic acidosis should be considered a sign of an underlying disease process. Identification of this underlying condition is essential for initiating prompt and appropriate treatment. Although symptoms can vary, people with metabolic acidosis often experience the following:

- Agitation
- Anxiety
- Confusion
- Fatigue
- Fruity-smelling breath (a classic symptom of diabetic ketoacidosis)
- Headache
- Lethargy
- Loss of appetite
- Nausea
- Nervousness
- Rapid heartbeat
- Shortness of breath
- Vomiting
- Weakness

If you are experiencing these symptoms, contact your doctor. Severe metabolic acidosis may require hospitalization.

Testing for Metabolic Acidosis

The following tests are generally used to determine high acid levels in the blood:

Anion gap. This test measures the chemical balance in the blood by comparing the numbers of positively and negatively charged particles, including sodium, chloride, and bicarbonate.

Arterial blood gases. This test measures the pH of the blood and the levels of oxygen and carbon dioxide in it.

Urine tests. These tests can reveal ketoacidosis, kidney problems, alcohol poisoning, and poisoning by aspirin, ethylene glycol (found in antifreeze), or methanol. People with diabetes can do an at-home urine test for ketones using over-the-counter test strips. Some blood sugar meters can also measure ketones in the blood.

Standard Treatment for Metabolic Acidosis
Treatment for metabolic acidosis varies depending on the cause of the condition. If the acid-alkaline balance isn't restored, bones, muscles, and the kidneys can be affected, and in severe cases, the condition can cause shock or death. Diabetic ketoacidosis can induce coma. Immediate medical attention is strongly encouraged. Common treatments include the following:
- Detoxification for alcohol, drug, or chemical poisoning
- Insulin for diabetic ketoacidosis
- Intravenous fluids
- Intravenous sodium bicarbonate
- Hospitalization

Prevention of Metabolic Acidosis
While it's not always possible to prevent an occurrence of metabolic acidosis, there are a few steps you can take to lessen the chances of it happening:
- Hydrate with plenty of water and nonalcoholic fluids. Urine should be clear or pale yellow.
- Limit alcohol consumption. Alcohol increases acid buildup and causes dehydration.
- Manage your diabetes (if you have it).
- Take medications as directed.

Alkalosis

The prevailing premise of the acid-alkaline diet is that a more alkaline environment in the body can better ward off disease. At the core of this premise is the belief that although the body can be too acidic, it can't be too alkaline. Alkalosis, however, is a very real medical condition, even though it may not be as common or as widely discussed in health circles as acidosis. Decreased levels of carbon dioxide (an acid) or increased levels of bicarbonate (a base) can make the body too alkaline, resulting in alkalosis, a condition that's the opposite of acidosis. The following are the different types of alkalosis that can occur:

Compensated alkalosis. When the body's acid-base balance returns to normal after a case of alkalosis but the bicarbonate and carbon dioxide levels remain abnormal, the condition is called compensated alkalosis.

Hypochloremic alkalosis. Hypochloremic alkalosis is caused by an extreme lack or loss of chloride from the body. Although very uncommon, this can occur with prolonged vomiting, diuretic therapy, or nasogastric tube suctioning.

Hypokalemic alkalosis. When the kidneys respond to an extreme lack or loss of potassium, hypokalemic alkalosis is the result. This can also occur from taking certain types of diuretics.

Metabolic alkalosis. Too much bicarbonate in the blood causes metabolic alkalosis. This condition can also be caused by certain kidney diseases.

Respiratory alkalosis. Low carbon dioxide levels in the blood can result in respiratory alkalosis. This can be attributed to one of the following:
- Being at a high altitude
- Fever
- Lack of oxygen
- Liver disease
- Lung disease, which causes faster breathing (hyperventilation)
- Salicylate poisoning

Symptoms of Alkalosis

Although symptoms can vary, people with alkalosis may experience any of the following:
- Coma
- Confusion
- Hand tremor
- Light-headedness
- Muscle twitching

- Nausea
- Numbness or tingling in the face, hands, or feet
- Prolonged muscle spasms (tetany)
- Stupor
- Vomiting

Testing for Alkalosis

If alkalosis is suspected, a health care provider will perform a physical examination and inquire about symptoms. Some of the possible laboratory tests that may be ordered include an arterial blood gas analysis and an electrolytes test, such as a basic metabolic panel to confirm alkalosis and determine whether it is respiratory or metabolic alkalosis. Additional tests may be necessary to determine the cause of the alkalosis, including urinalysis and a urine pH test.

Standard Treatment for Alkalosis

Treatment for alkalosis varies based on the cause of the condition. For alkalosis caused by hyperventilation, breathing into a paper bag will help the body retain more carbon dioxide, improving the alkalosis. If a person's oxygen level is low, it may be necessary to administer oxygen. Medicines may be needed to correct chemical losses (such as chloride and potassium). Health care providers will also monitor vital signs, including temperature, pulse, rate of breathing, and blood pressure.

Most cases of alkalosis respond well to treatment. If untreated or not treated properly, alkalosis could result in arrhythmia, coma, or electrolyte imbalance (such as hypokalemia). Contact your health care provider if you become confused, are unable to concentrate, or are unable to catch your breath. Go to the emergency room or call your local emergency number (such as 911) if you experience any of the following:

- Loss of consciousness
- Rapidly worsening symptoms of alkalosis
- Seizure
- Severe breathing difficulties

Prevention of Alkalosis

Although prevention depends on the cause of the alkalosis, most people with healthy kidneys and lungs do not experience serious alkalosis.

The Effects of pH on the Environment and Our Food

All life relies on having the appropriate pH levels both within living organisms and within the cells of those organisms. Life on Earth is also dependent on a tightly controlled pH level of soil and water. With the expansion of industrialization and an increase in carbon dioxide buildup over the past century, the pH of the ocean dropped from 8.2 to 8.1, negatively impacting marine life and threatening the collapse of the coral reefs. The pH of our soil has also been adversely affected. Soil pH influences the mineral content of the food that's grown in it because minerals act as buffers to balance pH. To obtain the greatest nutrient density and usability, soil should have a pH level between 6 and 7. Soil with a pH below 6 is acidic and may have decreased amounts of calcium and magnesium. Soil with a pH above 7 is alkaline and may result in chemically unavailable or decreased amounts of copper, iron, manganese, and zinc. Two of the most common soil inputs used to improve the pH in acidic soil are dolomite and animal manure.

Our diets over the last two hundred years have dramatically decreased in potassium compared to sodium and increased in chloride compared to bicarbonate. It is widely known that the diets of modern humans are generally poor in magnesium and potassium, low in fiber, and high in saturated fat, sugar, sodium, and chloride, especially when compared to preagricultural humans. Consequently, our modern way of eating may induce metabolic acidosis, which has been particularly evident in older populations. For example, a diet high in refined carbohydrates and animal protein creates an increased acid load in the body. Although this produces very little change in blood pH, it leads to many changes in urinary chemistry, including decreased magnesium levels and pH and increased urinary calcium, undissociated uric acid, and phosphate. These factors result in a higher risk for kidney stones.

The Effects of pH on Our Health

The pH of our body fluids can be disrupted by two main forces: the acid- or alkaline-forming effects of the foods we ingest and the acids we generate through the body's regular metabolic activities. Fortunately, the body has three major mechanisms to help maintain the blood's pH and prevent dietary, metabolic, and other factors from pushing it outside its normal 7.35 to 7.45 range. These mechanisms include the following:

1. Buffering systems
2. Exhalation of carbon dioxide
3. Elimination of hydrogen ions via the kidneys

The standard modern diet, rich in animal protein and highly processed foods, such as white flour products and white sugar, puts an increased acid load on the body. If a person spends years eating a poor diet that is mainly acid forming, some of the body's natural buffering systems will be overworked and could create undesirable changes in health.

Here is one example of how our buffering systems can be overtaxed and result in negative health consequences: In order to bring about pH homeostasis, calcium phosphate salts, which are structural components of bones and teeth, are circulated in the body and then released in the urine. If the body fluids are regularly exposed to large quantities of acid-forming foods and liquids, the body will draw upon its reserves of calcium phosphate in order to supply the phosphate buffering system so it can neutralize the acid-forming effects of the diet. Over time, this could lead to structural weakness of bones and teeth. Drawing on calcium phosphate reserves at a high rate can exacerbate the amount of calcium that is eliminated in urine. This is why a predominantly acid-forming diet can increase the risk of developing calcium-rich kidney stones. Because our buffering systems work around the clock to neutralize the acids formed from everyday metabolic activities, it makes sense to follow a diet that doesn't create an additional burden on these systems.

Animal protein, especially red meat, requires huge amounts of alkaline minerals for complete digestive processing. When the buffering system seeks the alkalinity needed to offset the acid load from the meat, it turns first to the minerals currently in the digestive tract. If it fails to find alkaline nourishment there, it draws on the calcium, magnesium, phosphorus, and potassium stored in our bones. This is where wholesome greens and other alkaline foods that are naturally packed with essential vitamins and minerals come into play. When we eat a diet that is abundant in plant-based nutrients, the body has no need to draw on the stored minerals in the bones. But when we don't consume a nutrient-rich diet, or when we overconsume foods that promote acidity in the body, then the body starts tapping the reservoir of our bone resources. In the short term this isn't an issue, but in the long run it can have serious consequences, not just for our bone health but for our overall health.

Be aware that some of the calcium loss in urine may be due to inadequate intestinal absorption. It's important to note that most people in northern climates are deficient in vitamin D and that adequate supplementation with vitamin D enhances intestinal absorption of calcium, magnesium, and phosphate. It's also worth mentioning that the high acid renal load caused by excess animal protein could potentially be offset with the ingestion of alkaline-rich supplements or high-alkaline foods, such as vegetables and fruits.

In addition to high-acid foods, the modern diet contains excessive amounts of sodium, the degree of which may be a predictor of hyperchloremic metabolic acidosis. There is also evidence that a diet high in sodium will exacerbate bone and muscle loss in the aging population. Furthermore, dietary sodium has been shown to result in hypertension and osteoporosis in women, whereas dietary potassium, which is sorely lacking in the modern diet, could help moderate these effects.

The aging process decreases muscle mass in both men and women, making elders more susceptible to falls and fractures. Current research has shown that a diet that includes foods rich in potassium, such as vegetables and fruits, and low in acid-producing foods, such as animal products and refined foods, helps to preserve muscle mass as we age. Conditions that result in chronic metabolic acidosis, such as chronic renal failure, accelerate the breakdown of skeletal muscle. Rebalancing acidosis (such as by alkaline supplementation or by following an alkalizing diet) could potentially help offset muscle wasting and retain muscle mass in people with ailments such as diabetic ketosis, chronic obstructive lung disease, and renal failure that create this chronic condition.

Alkaline diets result in a more alkaline urine pH and may also result in decreased calcium in the urine; however, this may not necessarily be reflective of total calcium balance because of other buffers, such as phosphate. There is currently no substantial evidence that an alkaline diet protects from osteoporosis. Nevertheless, evidence to date suggests that alkaline diets may result in a number of other relevant health benefits:

- Increased vegetable and fruit intake, such as with a high-alkaline diet, would improve the ratio of potassium to sodium and therefore may benefit bone health, decrease muscle wasting, and possibly mitigate other chronic diseases, such as hypertension and stroke.
- The increase in natural growth hormone from a high-alkaline diet may improve many outcomes for various conditions, from cardiovascular health to cognition to memory.
- An alkalizing diet provides an increase in intracellular magnesium, a mineral that's required for the function of many enzyme systems and to activate vitamin D.
- The alkalinity provided by a high-alkaline diet may result in added benefit for some chemotherapeutic agents that require a higher pH. Please note, however, that there is no scientific literature at this time establishing the benefit of an alkaline diet for the prevention of cancer.

For these reasons alone, it would be prudent to consider a more alkaline diet to prevent and reduce the many chronic diseases that are plaguing the human population.

The Theory Behind the Acid-Alkaline Diet

The notion that we should consume mostly alkaline foods was first proposed during the 1930s by Weston Andrew Price, a dentist from Cleveland, Ohio, known primarily for his theories on the relationship between nutrition, dental health, and physical health. Price traveled to remote regions of the world and discovered that the native people in those areas, whose diets consisted of unprocessed foods, had healthier teeth than his patients, who were eating large amounts of processed foods. From his observations, he concluded that poor dental health was the result of nutritional deficiencies.

Although Weston Price had advocated a vegetarian diet as the healthiest choice, the current leaders of the Weston Andrew Price Foundation, a relatively small nonprofit with a modest budget, have been very vocal in advocating a meat-centered, dairy-centered diet. Unfortunately, what they promote is woefully inaccurate, out-of-date dietary advice that is entirely out of step both with Price's original premise and modern nutritional science.

Today the acid-alkaline diet, which is mostly endorsed by health advocates and alternative-medicine practitioners, isn't a single dietary approach but rather a group of loosely related diets. These diets are based on the belief that certain foods can alter the pH of body fluids, including urine and blood, and can consequently create a more alkaline environment in the body that is beneficial for treating and even preventing illness and disease. The theory revolves around the idea that upsetting the delicate acid-alkaline balance in the body is a major contributor to chronic disease. As it turns out, modern medicine does, for the most part, back up this theory (as shown in the previous sections of this book). In addition, advocates of a high-alkaline diet as well as conventional medical practitioners agree that environmental factors and precipitating health conditions are the primary influences on how acidic or alkaline the body will be. However, supporters of the acid-alkaline diet diverge from conventional medicine by contending that food, rather than standard medical treatments and medications, is what should be used to regulate the body when the acid-alkaline levels become imbalanced. While in theory this sounds reasonable and appealing, the question that needs to be asked and answered is whether this is even possible, given what we know about human physiology.

Changing the Body's pH

The relationship between diet and acid-base homeostasis, or the regulation and stabilization of the acid-alkaline status of the body, has been studied for decades. Alternative health practitioners who support this dietary approach have largely focused on how what we eat affects the acidity of our urine, with the assumption that the pH of our urine accurately represents the pH of our body as a whole. However, pH levels vary throughout the body. While blood is slightly alkaline, with a pH between 7.35 and 7.45, the stomach is very acidic, with a pH of 3.5 or below, so it can break down food. The pH of our urine fluctuates, depending on what we eat, as this is how the body keeps the pH level of the blood steady.

Supporters of the acid-alkaline diet have traditionally advocated for the avoidance of meat, poultry, cheese, wheat and other grains, processed foods, and sugar to alkalinize (increase the pH) of urine. Indeed, there's some early evidence showing that a diet low in these acid-producing foods and high in vegetables and fruits, both of which are more alkaline, could help prevent kidney stones (nephrolithiasis) and recurrent urinary tract infections (UTIs), keep bones and muscles strong, improve heart health and brain function, decrease lower back pain, and reduce the risk for colon cancer and type 2 diabetes. In fact, acid-alkaline imbalance has been mentioned in various scientific publications as a potential risk factor for osteoporosis, but the available weight of the current scientific evidence does not support this hypothesis. Results of this dietary approach on osteoporosis prevention and treatment have, to date, been either ineffective or variable, and measurement of urine pH hasn't been a reliable predictor of bone fractures or loss of bone mineral density. This has led conventional health practitioners to recommend pharmaceuticals, rather than diet modification, as the preferred method of changing urine pH.

Table 1. pH of selected fluids, organs, and membranes

Organ, fluid, or membrane	Natural pH	Function of pH
Bile	7.6 to 8.8	Neutralizes stomach acid; aids digestion
Cerebrospinal fluid	7.3	Bathes the exterior of the brain
Gastric	1.35 to 3.5	Breaks down protein
Intracellular fluid	6.0 to 7.2	Attributable to acid production in cells
Pancreatic fluid	8.8	Neutralizes stomach acid; aids digestion
Serum arterial	7.4	Tightly regulated
Serum venous	7.35	Tightly regulated
Skin	4 to 6.5	Provides a protective barrier from microbes
Urine	4.6 to 8.0	Limits overgrowth of microbes
Vaginal fluid	<4.7	Limits overgrowth of opportunistic microbes

Source: *J Environ Public Health*. Published online Oct. 12, 2011. doi: 10.1155/2012/727630.

Proponents of the alkaline diet claim that it can help the body maintain its blood pH level. In reality, nothing we eat is going to substantially change the pH of the body's fluids. As noted earlier, the body has a variety of systems that work to keep the pH levels of blood and urine regulated and constant. Nevertheless, supporters of the alkaline diet say that although acid-producing foods shift the pH balance of blood or urine just briefly, if we keep shifting the pH over and over in the direction of acidity, we could be creating long-lasting acidosis that may be the root cause of many of our modern-day ills. Likewise, if we continually shift the body fluids toward an alkaline pH, we might reap the health benefits of a more alkalinized system.

The Acid-Alkaline Diet FAQs

What are the fundamentals of the acid-alkaline diet?
The standard American diet is highly acid forming, overwhelming the body's natural mechanisms for removing excess acid. The staples of the typical American diet, such as meat, dairy products, wheat, processed foods, and refined sugar, are acidifying. At the same time, the diet is notably deficient in alkalizing vegetables and fruits. Eating a high-alkaline diet can help mitigate this acid load, decreasing the strain on the body's acid-detoxification systems, particularly the kidneys.

The acid-alkaline diet emphasizes alkaline foods, such as whole fruits and vegetables and other plant foods. A balanced acid-alkaline diet includes both acidifying and alkalizing foods; however, the scales are tilted heavily toward the alkalizing foods. The body has a variety of systems that are adept at neutralizing and eliminating excess acid, but there is a limit to how heavy an acid load even a healthy body can effectively manage. The body is inherently capable of maintaining an acid-alkaline balance provided that the organs are healthy and functioning properly and that other acid-producing factors, such as tobacco use and high consumption of acidifying foods—including meat, sugar, refined carbohydrates, and other processed products—are minimized or completely avoided.

What does "alkaline forming" mean when it comes to food?
Alkaline-forming foods are those that might not necessarily be alkaline when tested but that produce an alkaline effect when ingested by the human body. For example, citrus fruits, such as lemons and grapefruits, which contain citric acid and taste sour, are alkalizing to the body once they're consumed.

What are the benefits of eating alkaline foods?

A high-alkaline diet might help to offset and neutralize excessive amounts of acid that can lead to inflammation and other chronic conditions. However, there is currently no scientific evidence that foods can actually change the pH level of the blood and therefore alter the way the body handles certain diseases and conditions. Nevertheless, alkaline foods tend to be those that are generally known to support health and well-being—fruits, vegetables, legumes, and whole grains. So it's possible that the acid-alkaline diet is simply health promoting overall because it includes nutrient-dense foods that are rich in antioxidants and phytochemicals while cutting out unhealthy foods.

Can alkaline foods benefit acid reflux?

The types of foods recommended on an alkalizing diet, such as fresh vegetables and fruits and lower-fat nuts, seeds, and legumes, tend to help lessen or prevent the symptoms of acid reflux. The foods avoided on an alkalizing diet are those that generally exacerbate the condition, such as high-fat foods, fried foods, oils, meats, sugar, and refined carbohydrates. It's always wise to ask your doctor for a diet plan that will lessen the symptoms of acid reflux, but you might find that what you're given is comparable to an acid-alkaline diet.

Do alkaline foods promote weight loss?

Although the acid-alkaline diet isn't a weight-loss regimen, it will likely encourage weight loss. That's because alkaline foods are generally low in fat and calories, high in protein and fiber, and nutrient dense, so you'll be able to ingest larger quantities of food but take in fewer calories, making you feel more satisfied after eating and keeping you feeling full longer.

How do alkaline foods taste?

The list of alkaline foods is extensive and varied, and there's no single taste to describe them. Many of these foods are vegetables, some are fruits, and some are nuts, legumes, or grains. Know that acid-producing foods (such as meat and sugar) don't actually taste acidic, but they have an acid-forming effect within the body. The flavor of a food doesn't provide a clue as to whether it's alkaline or acidic.

Does cooking food make it more acidic?
Cooking doesn't necessarily change the acidity or alkalinity of food, and it's not necessary to have an all-raw menu to follow a high-alkaline diet.

Can a high-alkaline diet prevent or treat cancer?
There have been no studies to date that have shown that a high-alkaline diet can prevent, treat, or reverse cancer. Although there are people who claim that eating acid-forming foods can lead to cancer and allow it to thrive and spread in the body, doctors and scientists will say that the body maintains the blood at a certain pH regardless of what we eat. If that's true, then you might ask what the point would be in encouraging cancer patients to eat a more alkaline diet. The fact is that the foods advocated by practitioners of the acid-alkaline diet happen to be those that are healthy, and the foods they encourage avoidance of happen to be those that are known to cause a variety of chronic diseases and that are also associated with greater cancer risk.

Can alkaline foods cure gout?
Gout is caused by an excessive amount of uric acid in the body. A high-alkaline diet may help offset and neutralize those acid levels and diminish gout attacks. Special diets designed for people with gout are very similar to the acid-alkaline plan, so by eating close to this diet style, people with gout will be avoiding many of the known foods that trigger gout attacks.

Can high-alkaline foods cure acne?
Not surprisingly, acid-forming foods, such as those that are sugary, fatty, and greasy, are associated with acne breakouts. The reason may not be that

the food is acid forming, however. It could be that diets laden with these types of foods are also devoid of the items advocated on a high-alkaline diet, which are foods rich in the vitamins, minerals, and antioxidants that promote healthy, blemish-free skin.

Is the acid-alkaline diet recommended for people with diabetes?
Because the acid-alkaline diet discourages eating sugar and processed foods, it may help people with diabetes keep their blood glucose levels in check so they don't get the types of spikes that typically follow eating high-sugar foods. For people who don't have diabetes, the chances of getting type 2 diabetes would likely be decreased on a high-alkaline diet. And for those who already have diabetes, the alkaline diet may help with symptom management. Be sure to consult with your doctor before starting an alkaline diet (or any diet) if you have diabetes.

Can alkaline foods cure other diseases and conditions?
There have been many claims that a high-alkaline diet can cure everything under the sun and that people are only susceptible to certain illnesses and diseases when their bodies are acidic. But what does it mean to say that a person's body is either alkaline or acidic? There are some parts of the body that need to be acidic in order to function properly. For example, we wouldn't want the stomach to be alkaline or it wouldn't be able to break down food. As food makes its way from the mouth to the stomach, the digestive tract becomes more acidic. Pepsin, the enzyme responsible for protein breakdown, needs an acidic environment, and therefore pepsin gets released into the stomach, where pH is very low (between 1.5 and 2.0). The small intestine is where most of the nutrients in food get absorbed and where the pH increases from 2.0 to 6.5 as the food travels from the stomach to the small and large intestines. The acidic environment of the stomach is not only necessary for processing food, but it also helps to protect the body from pathogenic organisms and harmful food antigens. In addition,

the body is going to regulate the blood's pH levels regardless of what we eat, the same way it keeps the heart beating, the lungs functioning, and certain organs and body parts at specific temperatures. If you have a health problem, consult with your doctor before fully subscribing to any diet plan, including an acid-alkaline diet.

Measuring the Acid and Alkaline Effects of Food

One of the most reliable measures of the acidic or basic effects foods have in the body is the potential renal acid load (PRAL). PRAL is a calculation method that estimates a food's potential to create acid or alkaline residue after it has been digested. Through this system of measurement, researchers are able to analyze a food and, based on its components, determine what the true acid or base load on the body will be. PRAL is a scientific approach based on a simple formula created by researchers Thomas Remer and Friedrich Manz. Their paper on this topic, "Potential renal acid load of foods and its influence on urine pH," was published in the *Journal of the American Dietetic Association* in July 1995 (95: 791-797). PRAL scores are broken down as follows:

• Foodstuffs with a negative PRAL value exert an alkaline effect.
• Foodstuffs with a positive PRAL value exert an acidic effect.
• Foodstuffs with a zero PRAL value have a neutral effect.

According to their calculation model, negative PRAL values (indicating an excess of the base-forming potential of foods) were nearly exclusively found in the vegetable and fruit groups. In contrast, the highest acid loads originated in cheese, followed by meat, fish, and grain products. More than one hundred frequently consumed foods and beverages were studied by Remer and Manz.

The research by Remer and Manz proved that only five substances in a food need to be measured to have a reliable estimate of the outcome after the food has been digested. These five substances include acid-producing and alkaline-producing material. It is vital that our diets include both types of foods, but the overall balance should lean heavily toward the alkaline side.

The United States Department of Agriculture (USDA) developed the PRAL formula with constants, which are determined by the amount of acid-neutralizing minerals found in urine. This formula can be used to calculate the approximate acidifying effects of the foods we eat based on the amounts of magnesium, phosphorus, protein, calcium, and potassium they contain. The concept of PRAL calculation is based on human physiology and takes into account the different intestinal absorption rates of individual minerals and of sulfur-containing proteins, as well as the amount of sulfate produced from metabolized proteins. Here is the basic formula: PRAL = 0.49 x (g) protein + 0.037 x (mg) phosphorus − 0.021 x (mg) potassium − 0.026 x (mg) magnesium − 0.013 x (mg) calcium.

Table 2. PRAL formula

PRAL Score =	Acid	0.49 x (g) protein + 0.037 x (mg) phosphorus
	Minus Alkaline	− 0.021 x (mg) potassium − 0.026 x (mg) magnesium − 0.013 x (mg) calcium

You can use this formula to evaluate the PRAL of any food product (processed or raw) as long as you can provide the required nutritional values per a 100 gram sample. A 100 gram sample is used as the standard to make it easier to compare various products. The USDA has calculated the values for thousands of foods we consume every day. To easily search items in this database, go to http://health-diet.us/lowaciddiet.

The following tables show the PRAL scores as drawn from the study by Remer and Manz.

Table 3. PRAL of meat and meat products per 100 grams

Meat Product	PRAL Score
Beef, lean	7.8
Chicken, meat only	8.7
Corned beef, canned	13.2
Frankfurter	6.7
Liver sausage	10.6
Luncheon meat, canned	10.2
Pork, lean	7.9
Rump steak, lean and fat	8.8
Salami	7.6
Turkey, meat only	9.9
Veal, fillet	9.0

Table 4. PRAL of fish per 100 grams

Fish	PRAL Score
Cod fillet	7.1
Haddock	6.8
Herring	7.0
Trout	10.8

Table 5. PRAL of milk, dairy products, and eggs per 100 grams

Milk, Dairy Products, and Eggs	PRAL Score
Buttermilk	0.5
Cheese, hard	19.2
Cheddar, low fat	26.4
Cottage cheese	8.7
Egg white	1.1
Egg yolk	23.4

Gouda cheese	18.6
Ice cream	0.6
Parmesan cheese	34.2
Processed cheese	28.7
Sour cream	1.2
Whole egg	8.2
Whole milk	1.1
Whole milk, pasteurized	0.7
Whole milk yogurt, plain	1.5
Whole milk yogurt, with fruit	1.2

Table 6. PRAL of sugar and sweets per 100 grams

Sugar and Sweets	PRAL Score
Cake	3.7
Honey	−0.3
Marmalade	−1.5
Milk chocolate	2.4
Sugar, white	−0.1

Table 7. PRAL of vegetables per 100 grams

Vegetables	PRAL Score
Asparagus	−0.4
Broccoli	−1.2
Carrot	−4.9
Cauliflower	−4.0
Celery	−5.2
Chicory	−2.0
Cucumber	−0.8
Eggplant	−3.4

Leek	−1.8
Lettuce	−2.5
Mushroom	−1.4
Onion	−1.5
Pepper (Capsicum)	−2.8
Potato	−3.1
Radish	−2.6
Spinach	−14.0
Tomato	−3.1
Tomato juice	−2.8
Zucchini	−2.6

Table 8. PRAL of fruits, nuts, and juices per 100 grams

Fruits, Nuts, and Juices	**PRAL Score**
Apple	−2.2
Apple juice	−2.2
Apricot	−4.8
Banana	−5.5
Black currants	−6.5
Cherries	−3.6
Grape juice	−1.0
Hazelnuts	−2.8
Kiwifruit	−4.1
Lemon juice	−2.5
Orange	−2.7
Orange juice	−2.9
Peach	−2.4
Peanuts	8.3
Pear	−2.9

Pineapple	−2.7
Raisins	−21.0
Strawberries	−2.2
Walnuts	6.8
Watermelon	−1.9

Table 9. PRAL of grain products per 100 grams

Grain Products	PRAL Score
Cornflakes	6.0
Crackers, rye	3.3
Noodles, egg	6.4
Oats	10.7
Rice, brown	12.5
Rice, white	1.7
Rye bread	4.1
Rye bread, mixed grain	4.0
Rye flour	5.9
Spaghetti, white	6.5
Spaghetti, whole grain	7.3
Wheat bread	1.8
Wheat bread, mixed grain	3.8
White bread	3.7
Wheat flour	8.2

Table 10. PRAL of legumes per 100 grams

Legumes	PRAL Score
Green beans	−3.1
Lentils	3.5
Peas	1.2

Table 11. PRAL of fats and oils per 100 grams

Fats and Oils	PRAL Score
Butter	0.6
Margarine	0.5
Olive oil	0.0
Sunflower oil	0.0

Table 12. PRAL of beverages per 100 grams

Beverages	PRAL Score
Beer, draft	−0.2
Beer, pale	0.9
Beer, stout	−0.1
Coca Cola	0.4
Cocoa	−0.4
Coffee	−1.4
Mineral water	−1.8
Tea	−0.3
Wine, red	−2.4
Wine, white	−1.2

Table 13. Average PRAL score for various food groups

Food Groups	Average PRAL Score
Beverages	
Alkali rich	−1.7
Alkali poor	0
Dairy products and cheese	
Milk and non-cheese	1.0
Low-protein cheese	8.0
High-protein cheese	23.6

Fats and oils	0
Fish	7.9
Fruits, nuts, and juices	−3.1
Grain products	
Bread	3.5
Flour	7.0
Noodles	6.7
Legumes	1.2
Meat and meat products	9.5
Sugar and sweets	4.3
Vegetables	−2.8

Calculating the PRAL Score for a Meal

From the PRAL tables shown on pages 25 to 30, it's evident that the standard American diet, with its emphasis on excessive intakes of animal protein, produces an extremely heavy acid load. You can use these tables to help calculate the PRAL score for each of your meals. Here's how:

1. Record the amount in grams of each food you eat in a meal.
2. Multiply the PRAL score in the tables by your food amount.

Table 14. PRAL calculation for a sample meal of lentils, potato, and spinach

Food	Amount	PRAL per 100 grams	PRAL Calculation	PRAL Score
Lentils	198 grams (1 cup)	3.1	3.1 x 1.98	6.14
Potato	250 grams (8 ounces)	−4.0	−.40 x 2.5	−10.0
Spinach	100 grams (3.5 ounces)	−14.0	−14.0 x 1.0	−14.0
TOTAL PRAL				−17.86

For the sample meal in table 14 (page 30) the tally is 6.14 for the lentils, −10.0 for the potato, and −14.0 for the spinach, for a total PRAL score of −17.86 for the meal. The alkalinity of the potato and spinach cancel out the slightly acidic score of the lentils, demonstrating how incorporating more vegetables and fruits at every meal can benefit the overall acid-alkaline ratio of the diet. Of course, centering a meal around plant proteins rather than animal proteins, along with including large amounts of fresh vegetables and fruits, will naturally keep the PRAL scores of meals deep in the alkaline range without any planning, effort, or calculations needed.

Improve Your pH Balance Naturally

Proponents of the acid-alkaline diet might tout the belief that just by eating high-alkaline food and avoiding acid-producing food we can achieve good health. While it's true that a healthy body maintains balance on its own as long as it receives proper nourishment, exercise, and rest, it's unrealistic and not scientifically sound to think that simply by loading up on alkalizing foods and supplements that medically diagnosed acidosis and related health problems could be corrected. To restore pH balance, other sources of metabolic acidity must also be addressed, because for most people, no amount of alkalizing through diet alone can reverse and balance a toxically acidic environment. In addition, detoxification and rebalancing pH happen gradually. Nevertheless, improving the alkalinity of our diets can, of course, benefit health, because alkaline foods are nutrient dense, packed with potent antioxidants and phytochemicals, low in calories and fat, and rich in fiber. In addition, they taste delicious and are inexpensive compared with refined and processed foods. They also are the foods most lacking in the standard American diet.

Start with Diet

The first place to begin when aiming for greater acid-alkaline equilibrium is with diet. Following are a few suggestions for how to restore pH balance to your diet, improve digestion, get blood pH levels back on track and help keep them stabilized, and protect your bones and kidneys in the process.

Load up on fresh vegetables, especially dark leafy greens. Dark leafy greens, such as chard, collards, kale, mustard greens, and spinach are particularly alkalizing. Accent them with freshly squeezed lemon or lime juice, both of which are also highly alkalizing.

Enjoy fresh fruits. Fruits with a low glycemic index that are deeply pigmented or brightly colored are the most beneficial.

Choose root vegetables. Root veggies, such as carrots, onions, parsnips, rutabagas, sweet potatoes, and turnips, are excellent sources of alkalizing mineral compounds.

Indulge in green superfoods. Green superfoods are those that are abundant in chlorophyll, which is a natural detoxifier and immunity builder. Foods that contain high levels of chlorophyll include the algae spirulina and chlorella and the juice of wheatgrass and other sprouted grains. These foods are also rich in antioxidants and micronutrients.

Enjoy green smoothies. Adding tender dark leafy greens to smoothies that are based on alkalizing fruits is a delicious and simple way to increase your intake of alkaline foods.

Eat plenty of vegetable protein. Most people would be surprised to know that virtually all plants contain protein. Tempeh, tofu, and millet are particularly alkalizing.

Focus on whole grains. When you include grains in your diet, select those that are whole, with the bran intact, such as brown rice, millet, quinoa, and wild rice.

Avoid animal protein. Animal protein includes chicken, dairy products (butter, cheese, milk, and yogurt), eggs, fish, pork, red meat, and anything that is made from or comes out of an animal's body.

Eliminate all processed foods. Processed foods include anything that's been refined, particularly products that contain white flour and sugar, are high in fat or have been fried, or have unpronounceable or multisyllabic words in the ingredient list. Instead of buying processed foods, purchase fresh foods that don't come in a package and don't contain any ingredients other than what nature provided.

Additional Steps

Being healthy means not only focusing on diet and choosing nutritious foods but also improving other areas of life. We all know that getting sufficient exercise and sleep, doing meaningful work, and having supportive, rewarding relationships can benefit both our emotional and physical well-being. Here are a few more easy-to-implement things you can do to improve the quality of your health.

Hydrate. The majority of people don't drink enough water and are chronically dehydrated, which has a negative effect on energy, immunity, health, and overall quality of life. Filter your water and aim to drink between six and eighteen cups of water per day. One way to improve the alkalinity of your water is to add freshly squeezed lemon juice to it. To make lemon water, add ¼ cup of lemon juice to 2 cups of lukewarm filtered water. Another enjoyable way to hydrate is with organic, caffeine-free herbal teas (with no sugar added).

Transition slowly. Take your time transitioning to a more alkaline diet and healthy lifestyle. Don't try to do everything at once. Experiment with finding alkalizing foods that you and your family like. Have fun creating new meal plans that work for you for the long term. Look at your lifestyle changes as expansive rather than restrictive.

Breathe. Simple breathing exercises, performed once or twice a day, will go a long way with helping your body remove excess acid. Even if you just take the time to sit, focus your mind, visualize, and relax, you'll be improving your acid-alkaline balance.

Supplement. Green powder, which is a combination of powdered whole grasses, fruits, vegetables, and sprouts (with an emphasis on wheatgrass and barley grass) is a highly alkalizing supplement. Check out green powders from Aloha (aloha.com), Amazing Grass (amazinggrass.com), and

Garden of Life (gardenoflife.com), as well as other reliable brands. Alkaline water can be made using a water ionizer, pH drops, or adding freshly squeezed lemon juice (see "Hydrate," page 33) to filtered water. Supplementing with alkaline minerals, such as calcium, magnesium, potassium, and sodium, can help the body buffer acids.

Alkalizing Foods

While there is a plethora of conflicting information on the web regarding which foods are alkaline and which are acid forming, the easiest rule of thumb is to simply focus on foods you already know are good for you: fresh vegetables, salads, dark leafy greens, low-sugar fruits, nuts, and seeds, with an emphasis on unrefined, organic foods with a high water content. Aim for a ratio of 80:20; that is, try to make about 80 percent of your diet alkaline foods with the remaining 20 percent acidic foods. That said, know that eating a high percentage of alkaline foods will naturally offset any acidic foods you consume, and if your diet is primarily or completely based on plant foods, you don't need to be meticulous about this percentage, especially if you're eating a large quantity of whole, unadulterated vegetables and fruits. The aim is to keep the PRAL score (see page 24) of each meal and the overall PRAL score for the day deep in the negative (alkaline) values.

The following food groups are generally considered very alkalizing, so feel free to choose from them liberally:

- Fresh herbs (such as basil, cilantro, garlic, and parsley)
- Grasses (such as barley grass and wheatgrass)
- Green leafy vegetables (such as collard greens, kale, and spinach)
- Sea vegetables (such as blue-green algae, dulse, kelp, nori, and spirulina)
- Sprouts (such as alfalfa, mung bean, soybean, and sunflower)
- Medicinal mushrooms (such as maitake, reishi, and shiitake)
- Wild edibles (such as dandelion leaves and roots, nettles, and wild grasses)

Conclusion

The pH of the body will vary greatly depending on which part of the body is being referenced. A healthy body will naturally regulate the pH of its various systems so that each one stays at the optimum level for that particular bodily environment. The blood maintains a specific pH range and that range isn't directly affected by the foods we eat. The pH of urine, however, will vary depending on what we consume and our age, health, and nutrient absorption capabilities.

Food can be acidic, alkaline, or neutral. An excess of acidic foods will increase the body's acid load, causing mineral losses through urine. These losses could potentially be related to chronic or degenerative diseases, but no definitive scientific correlation has yet been confirmed through evidence-based research. Nevertheless, studies have shown that alkaline foods will help balance a diet-induced acid burden. However, the ideal objective is to eat a primarily alkaline diet that will help avoid any toxic acidic overload in the first place. The easiest and most effective way to do that is by following a diet based primarily or, better yet, solely on plant foods.

Alkalizing Recipes

Toasted Pumpkin or Sunflower Seeds

Makes ½ cup

Alkalizing pumpkin and sunflower seeds add extra flavor and crunch when sprinkled over salads, steamed vegetables, or whole grains. They're also great for a simple, quick snack on the go.

- ½ cup raw pumpkin seeds or sunflower seeds
- 2 teaspoons reduced-sodium tamari

Put the seeds in a medium skillet and toast over medium heat, stirring almost constantly, until fragrant and lightly browned, about 5 minutes. Pumpkin seeds will make popping sounds when they're perfectly toasted. Remove from the heat. Sprinkle with the tamari and stir rapidly until the seeds are evenly coated. Immediately transfer to a plate to cool.

Refreshing Cucumber Smoothie

Makes 2 servings

This potent smoothie will energize you for the entire day. Enjoy it for breakfast or lunch or anytime you need a power-packed treat loaded with alkalizing greens.

> 1 ripe avocado, cut into chunks
> Juice of 1 lemon
> 1 cucumber, coarsely chopped
> 2 stalks celery, coarsely chopped
> 2 cups spinach leaves or baby spinach, lightly packed
> ½ cup coarsely chopped fresh parsley, lightly packed
> 10 ice cubes made with filtered water

Put all the ingredients in a high-speed blender in the order listed and process on high speed until smooth.

Sweet Green Smoothie

Makes 2 servings

This smoothie is so rich and satisfying that you could even serve it for a light lunch or supper.

> 1 banana, frozen and broken into chunks
> 1 pear, cut into chunks (peeling optional)
> 2 cups spinach leaves or baby spinach, lightly packed, or 5 stemmed kale leaves
> 2½ cups filtered water
> ⅓ cup almond butter
> 1 teaspoon vanilla extract
> ½ teaspoon ground cinnamon

Put all the ingredients in a high-speed blender in the order listed and process on high speed until smooth.

Banana-Strawberry Smoothie

Makes 2 servings

This basic smoothie is a go-to staple. It's a smart idea to always keep frozen bananas and strawberries on hand so you can make this wholesome, naturally smoothie whenever the mood strikes.

> 2 ripe bananas, frozen and broken into chunks
> 1 cup frozen strawberries
> 2 stalks celery, sliced
> 5 pitted soft dates
> 2 cups filtered water

Put all the ingredients in a high-speed blender in the order listed and process on high speed until smooth.

Breakfast Quinoa

Makes 2 servings

If you have leftover quinoa in the fridge, you can whip up this tasty, high-protein breakfast lickety-split. It will fill you up and sustain you for hours without weighing you down.

> 1½ cups cooked quinoa (see Go-To Quinoa, page 44)
> 1½ cups plain or vanilla almond milk or other nondairy milk
> 3 tablespoons raw sunflower seeds or pumpkin seeds
> 3 tablespoons chopped dried apricots
> 3 tablespoons dried cranberries
> 1 tablespoon pure maple syrup (optional)
> ½ teaspoon ground cinnamon

Put all the ingredients in a medium saucepan and bring to a simmer over medium-high heat. Decrease the heat to medium and cook, stirring frequently, until the quinoa has absorbed most of the liquid and the dried fruit has plumped, about 10 minutes.

Spelt Porridge

Makes 1 serving

Spelt, an ancient relative of wheat, has never been hybridized and is more easily digested than other forms of wheat. Many people with wheat sensitivities find they're able to tolerate spelt. However, spelt is not gluten-free, so if you have celiac disease or gluten intolerance, you'll need to avoid it. High in fiber and a good source of iron and manganese, rolled spelt flakes can replace rolled oats in any recipe you want to make more alkaline.

- 1¼ cups filtered water, plus more as needed
- ⅓ cup rolled spelt flakes
- ¼ teaspoon vanilla extract
- Dash ground cinnamon (optional)
- ¼ cup fresh blueberries, blackberries, or sliced strawberries
- 1 tablespoon sliced almonds
- ½ cup plain or vanilla almond milk or other nondairy milk
- Pure maple syrup (optional)

Put the water, spelt flakes, vanilla extract, and optional cinnamon in a small saucepan and bring to a boil over high heat. Decrease the heat to low, cover, and cook, stirring frequently, until thick and creamy, 15 to 20 minutes. If the mixture becomes too dry or thick, add more water as desired. Spoon into a deep bowl and top with the blueberries, almonds, and almond milk. If desired, sweeten to taste with maple syrup.

Tip: For a creamier porridge, soak the spelt flakes in the water directly in the saucepan for 10 minutes before cooking. Thin spelt flakes will cook faster than thick ones, so adjust the cooking time and amount of liquid as necessary depending on the thickness of the spelt flakes.

Quinoa-Coconut Granola Bars

Makes 6 bars

These slightly sweet, high-protein granola bars are filling, alkalizing, and perfect for breakfast or a snack on the run. Plus, they're gluten-free and don't require any baking. What could be better?

> ⅔ cup sunflower seed butter or almond butter
> 3 tablespoons pure maple syrup
> 1 teaspoon vanilla extract
> ½ teaspoon ground cinnamon
> 1 cup quinoa flakes
> ⅓ cup unsweetened shredded dried coconut
> 2 tablespoons currants, raisins, dried cherries, or dried cranberries

Line an 8 x 4-inch loaf pan with parchment paper.

Put the sunflower seed butter, maple syrup, vanilla extract, and cinnamon in a medium bowl. Stir until smooth and well combined. Add the quinoa flakes, coconut, and currants. Stir until well combined, using your hands if necessary. The mixture will be thick and dry but should stick together.

Press the mixture firmly and evenly into the lined loaf pan. Refrigerate for at least 2 hours before serving. To slice, lift out of the pan using the parchment paper and cut crosswise into bars. Tightly wrap leftovers and store in the refrigerator.

Mango, Cucumber, and Quinoa Salad

Makes 4 servings

Naturally sweet and savory, this refreshing, light, and crunchy salad pleases almost every palate.

- 4 cups cooked quinoa (see Go-To Quinoa, page 44), cooled to room temperature
- 1 ripe mango, diced
- 1 small English cucumber, diced
- ¼ cup slivered almonds
- 2 tablespoons raw or toasted (see page 35) pumpkin seeds
- 2 tablespoons chopped fresh cilantro or parsley
- 2 tablespoons extra-virgin olive oil
- Juice of 1 lime
- Sea salt
- Freshly ground black pepper

Put the quinoa, mango, cucumber, almonds, pumpkin seeds, cilantro, oil, and lime juice in a large bowl and toss gently. Season with salt and pepper to taste and toss gently again. Serve immediately.

White Bean Stew

Makes 4 servings

This hearty stew comes together quickly if you have cooked or canned white beans on hand. It makes a great meal starter for four people, or it can serve as the main course for two.

- 4 cups filtered water
- 3 cups cooked or canned white beans (such as cannellini or great Northern beans), drained
- ½ head green cabbage, chopped
- 1 small onion, chopped
- 1 small potato, chopped (peeling optional)
- 1 carrot, chopped (peeling optional)
- 3 cloves garlic, minced
- 1 teaspoon ground fennel
- 1 teaspoon dried rosemary
- 1 teaspoon dried thyme
- 1 bay leaf
- ½ cup chopped fresh parsley, lightly packed
- Sea salt
- Freshly ground black pepper

Put the water, beans, cabbage, onion, potato, carrot, garlic, fennel, rosemary, thyme, and bay leaf in a large soup pot and bring to a boil over high heat. Decrease the heat to medium-low, partially cover, and cook, stirring occasionally, until the vegetables are tender, about 40 minutes. Remove the bay leaf.

Put half the soup in a blender and process until smooth. Pour the blended mixture back into the soup pot. Reheat if necessary. Stir in the parsley and season with salt and pepper to taste.

Kale and Sweet Potato Burritos

Makes 2 servings

Kale and sweet potatoes are a beautiful combination, and they're as delicious to eat as they are lovely to look at. When kale, sweet potatoes, and lentils are mixed with alkalizing quinoa, the result is some very satisfying eating.

> 1 sweet potato, peeled and diced
>
> 4 cups stemmed and chopped kale, lightly packed
>
> 1 cup cooked quinoa (see Go-To Quinoa, page 44)
>
> ½ cup cooked or canned lentils, drained
>
> 1 tablespoon balsamic vinegar
>
> ½ teaspoon ground cumin
>
> ½ teaspoon dried oregano
>
> 2 brown rice tortillas
>
> 1 small, ripe avocado, mashed
>
> Freshly squeezed lime or lemon juice

Steam the sweet potato for 5 minutes. Add the kale and steam for 5 minutes longer, or until the sweet potato is soft.

Put the quinoa, lentils, vinegar, cumin, and oregano in a medium bowl. Add the sweet potato and kale and stir gently to combine.

Warm the tortillas in a large skillet (preferably nonstick) until soft and pliable but not crispy, 2 to 3 minutes, turning them over once. Transfer the tortillas to a flat surface. Spread each tortilla with half the avocado. Sprinkle with lime juice as desired. Top with the quinoa mixture. Fold in the sides of the tortillas, then roll them up tightly from the bottom, pushing in any filling that escapes. With the folded side facing down, cut the burritos in half on the diagonal.

Curried Tofu and Veggie Stir-Fry

Makes 4 servings

This alkalizing stir-fry is a great dinner staple, and leftovers make a welcome lunch. For an even more filling dish, serve the stir-fry over cooked quinoa, brown rice, wild rice, or brown rice pasta. Feel free to change up the vegetables with your favorites.

- 1 pound extra-firm tofu, cut into 2 x 1-inch strips
- 1 tablespoon reduced-sodium tamari
- 1 tablespoon coconut oil
- ¼ cup raw or toasted (see page 35) pumpkins seeds
- 1 tablespoon peeled and minced fresh ginger
- ½ jalapeño chile, seeded and minced
- 2 cloves garlic, minced
- 1 large carrot, peeled and thinly sliced on the diagonal
- 1 head baby bok choy, rinsed and sliced crosswise on the diagonal
- 2 small zucchini, halved lengthwise and thinly sliced on the diagonal
- 1 tablespoon curry powder
- 1 cup full-fat or lite coconut milk
- ¼ cup chopped fresh cilantro or parsley, lightly packed
- Sea salt

Put the tofu in a medium bowl, sprinkle with the tamari, and toss gently to coat.

Heat the oil in a large skillet over medium-high heat. Add the pumpkin seeds, ginger, chile, and garlic and stir to combine. Add the carrot and cook, stirring frequently, until slightly softened, about 5 minutes. Add the bok choy and zucchini and cook, stirring frequently, until all the vegetables are tender. Add the curry powder and stir to combine. Stir in the tofu, coconut milk, and cilantro. Season with salt to taste. Decrease the heat to low, cover, and cook, stirring occasionally, until heated through and the flavors have blended, about 5 minutes.

Go-To Quinoa

Makes 4 cups

Alkalizing, gluten-free, nutrient-rich quinoa (pronounced KEEN-wah) makes a terrific replacement for rice, bulgur, couscous, millet, or pasta. Technically not a grain but an herb, quinoa was a staple food of the Incas of Peru. With its mild flavor and pleasing texture, quinoa works beautifully as an ingredient in salads and soups, as a side dish, or as a hearty main dish when combined with vegetables and beans. Containing all nine essential amino acids, quinoa is a complete protein and a versatile superfood.

> 1 cup quinoa (see tip)
> 2 cups filtered water

Put the quinoa in a medium saucepan. Add the water and bring to a boil over medium-high heat. Decrease the heat to low, cover, and cook undisturbed until all the water is absorbed, 25 to 30 minutes. The quinoa is done when the grain appears soft and translucent and the germ ring is visible along the outside of the grain.

Tip: If the quinoa you purchase isn't prerinsed (the package label should state if it is), put it in a fine-mesh strainer and rinse it well under running water, stirring it with your fingers, before using. Rinsing quinoa will remove its naturally occurring but bitter-tasting coating.

Coconut-Herb Sauce

Makes ⅔ cup

This rich, creamy sauce takes under five minutes to make, but the flavor is surprisingly complex. Drizzle it over your favorite steamed vegetables, cooked whole grains, or baked sweet potatoes, or use it as a salad dressing.

> ½ cup full-fat coconut milk
> 2 tablespoons chopped fresh dill, basil, or cilantro
> 1 tablespoon freshly squeezed lime or lemon juice
> Pinch ground turmeric
> Pinch sea salt
> Pinch freshly ground black pepper

Put all the ingredients in a small bowl and whisk until well combined. Cover and refrigerate for at least 1 hour before serving to allow the flavors to blend.

Mushrooms and Spinach

Makes 4 servings

This simple, two-vegetable combo makes a tempting side to accompany any savory dish.

> 2 tablespoons extra-virgin olive oil
> 1 pound mixed mushrooms, tough stems removed, sliced
> 4 cloves garlic, minced
> 1 teaspoon salt-free herb blend or Italian seasoning
> 2 cups baby spinach, firmly packed
> Sea salt
> Freshly ground black pepper

Put the oil in a large skillet and heat over medium-high heat. Add the mushrooms and stir to coat with the oil. Cover, decrease the heat to medium-low, and cook, stirring occasionally, for 5 minutes. Add the garlic and herb blend, cover, and cook, stirring occasionally, until the mushrooms are tender and most of the liquid has evaporated, about 5 minutes. Add the spinach and stir until wilted, 1 to 2 minutes. Season with salt and pepper to taste.

White Beans and Greens

Makes 4 servings

This traditional Italian dish is soothing and filling. It's packed with wholesome plant protein and alkalizing kale. You could also use Swiss chard or spinach in place of the kale if you prefer. To turn this side dish into a main dish, serve it over or alongside polenta, pasta, potatoes, or your favorite whole grain.

- 1 tablespoon extra-virgin olive oil
- 1 small onion, diced
- 2 cloves garlic, minced
- 5 cups stemmed and chopped kale, firmly packed
- ½ cup filtered water, plus more as needed
- 3 cups cooked or canned white beans (such as cannellini or great Northern beans), drained
- Sea salt
- Freshly ground black pepper

Heat the oil in a large skillet (preferably nonstick) over medium heat. Add the onion and garlic and cook, stirring frequently, until the onion is soft, about 5 minutes. Add the kale and water, cover, and cook, stirring occasionally, until the kale is wilted and tender to your liking, 5 to 10 minutes. If the kale is sticking, add a little more water as needed. Add the beans and stir until evenly distributed. Cover and cook, stirring occasionally, until the beans are heated through, 3 to 5 minutes. Season with salt and pepper to taste.

Eat-a-Rainbow Fruit Salad

Makes 4 servings

Fruit salad is light, refreshing, and alkalizing. It makes a delectable meal any time of the day or even a sweet dessert. To preserve the beautiful colors and full array of nutrients, prepare it just before serving.

- ½ cantaloupe, cut into bite-sized pieces
- 2 peaches or nectarines, cut into bite-sized pieces (peeling optional)
- 2 bananas, sliced
- 1 cup seedless green grapes, halved lengthwise
- 1 cup seedless red or purple grapes, halved lengthwise
- ½ cup sliced almonds
- 1 tablespoon freshly squeezed lime or lemon juice

Put all the ingredients in a large bowl and toss gently to combine.

Berry Good Fruit Salad

Makes 4 servings

Alkalizing berries are packed with health-protecting phytochemicals and are one of nature's most delicious superfoods.

- 2 nectarines, cut into bite-sized pieces (peeling optional)
- 1 pint blueberries
- 1 pint strawberries, hulled and halved or sliced
- 2 bananas, sliced
- 1 tablespoon freshly squeezed lime or lemon juice

Put all the ingredients in a large bowl and toss gently to combine.

About the Author

Jo Stepaniak is the author and coauthor of more than twenty books on food, health, and related lifestyle issues. She has dealt with multiple food sensitivities and understands firsthand the direct correlation between diet and wellness.

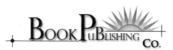

books that educate, inspire, and empower

All titles in the **Live Healthy Now** series are only **$5.95!**

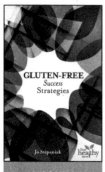 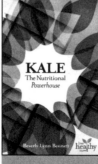 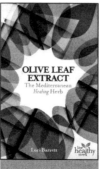 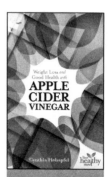

HEALTH ISSUES	HEALTHY FOODS	HERBS AND SUPPLEMENTS	NATURAL SOLUTIONS
A Holistic Approach to **ADHD**	Enhance Your Health with **FERMENTED FOODS**	**AROMATHERAPY** Essential Oils for Healing	Healthy and Beautiful with **COCONUT OIL**
Understanding **GOUT**	**GREEN SMOOTHIES** The Easy Way to Get Your Greens	The Pure Power of **MACA**	The Weekend **DETOX**
WHEAT BELLY Is Modern Wheat Causing Modern Ills?	**PALEO** Smoothies		Improve Digestion with **FOOD COMBINING**
	Refreshing Fruit and Vegetable **SMOOTHIES**		The Healing Power of **TURMERIC**

Interested in other health topics or healthy cookbooks? See our complete line of titles at **BookPubCo.com** or order directly from:
Book Publishing Company • PO Box 99 • Summertown, TN 38483 • 1-888-260-8458